What To Do When You're Expecting

10 Tips You Must Know As An Expecting Mother

By

Dr. Rebecca T. Luna

Table of Contents

INTRODUCTION

A woman's pregnancy is an exciting and transformational time, full of new experiences, difficulties, and joys. However, there is a lot of information and guidance available, which can make things confusing and overwhelming. It's critical for expectant mothers to take c[1]are of both themselves and their developing children and to be knowledgeable about the best procedures for a successful pregnancy and delivery.

This is the reason we created the document "What to Do When You're Expecting: 10 Tips You Must Know as an Expecting Mother." We'll give you all the advice you need in this manual to help you

---

[1]

confidently navigate pregnancy and motherhood.
We'll go through crucial subjects like:

Prenatal checkup appointments: We'll go over why routine prenatal exams are so crucial, what to expect during these visits, and how to pick the best healthcare provider for you.
Eating a balanced and nutritious diet: We'll go over the foods you should eat and stay away from while pregnant, as well as how to deal with typical pregnancy-related food issues including nausea and food aversions.

Staying hydrated: We'll go through the benefits of staying hydrated during pregnancy and provide advice on how to do so.

Regular exercise: We'll talk about the advantages of exercise during pregnancy as well as practical and secure strategies to keep active.

Getting enough rest and sleep is important throughout pregnancy. We'll offer advice on how to do this as well as solutions for common sleep issues including insomnia and frequent urination.

Avoiding alcohol, tobacco, and drugs: We'll discuss why it's crucial to abstain from these substances while pregnant and provide advice on how to do so if you're having trouble.

Prenatal vitamin use: We'll talk about the value of prenatal vitamins for a healthy pregnancy and provide advice on how to pick and use the best supplements.

Self-education on childbirth and parenting: We'll talk about how important it is to be knowledgeable and ready for both childbirth and motherhood and provide resources for more information.

Getting ready for your baby's arrival: We'll provide advice on cleaning up your house, picking a paediatrician, and making arrangements for your baby's postpartum care.

Reaching out to your support network: In this section, we'll talk about the value of having a strong support system during pregnancy and motherhood and provide advice on how to get in touch with friends, family, and other resources.

You'll be well on your way to a healthy and joyful pregnancy and parenting by paying attention to these ten suggestions. We hope that this guide will give you the knowledge and encouragement you require to fully enjoy this life-changing and exciting period.

CHAPTER ONE

Include Intensive Scheduling Of Prenatal Visits

Regular prenatal visits with your doctor are crucial to a healthy pregnancy and a safe birth when you're expecting a child. These sessions allow you the chance to keep an eye on your well-being and the development of your child while also getting advice and support from a medical expert.

Your doctor will likely conduct several tests and examinations during your prenatal visits to keep track of both your health and the growth of your unborn child. These may consist of:

Blood pressure checks: Preeclampsia, a dangerous pregnancy condition requiring medical intervention, can be detected by high blood pressure.

Urine tests: These exams can find conditions that could harm your unborn child, including urinary tract infections.

Blood tests: These checks can check for gestational diabetes, anaemia, and other potential health issues.

Ultrasound scans: An ultrasound can be performed to check for any anomalies, monitor the baby's growth and development, and confirm your due date.

Pelvic examinations: These examinations might find any problems that might harm your pregnancy, such as cervical alterations.

Your doctor will probably also inquire about your general health and any symptoms you may be having, such as nausea, exhaustion, or mood swings. They might share knowledge on birthing and parenting as well as suggestions for maintaining a balanced diet and exercising regularly.

Even if you feel OK and have no obvious health issues, it's crucial to go to all of your planned prenatal exams. To identify potential problems early and avoid complications later in your pregnancy, regular monitoring is essential.

During your appointments, don't be afraid to discuss any worries or inquiries you may have regarding your pregnancy with your healthcare provider. They are there to help you and make sure your pregnancy and birth are both healthy and enjoyable experiences.

You can take certain actions to make sure you get the most out of each appointment in addition to going to your prenatal checks. These consist of:

✓Arriving on time is crucial because

prenatal checks can take a while.

Make sure you arrive at your

appointment early

carrying a list of inquiries Before your visit, make a list of any queries or worries you may have so that you don't forget to bring them up.

✓Bringing a support person: Going to appointments with a spouse, family member, or friend can make you feel more

at ease and help you remember crucial details.

✓Keeping a journal of your symptoms will help you communicate with your healthcare practitioner about any changes in your symptoms or any new symptoms you may be experiencing.

✓Being open and honest about your habits: If you smoke, use drugs, or consume alcohol, let your healthcare professional know so they can offer the right advice and assistance.

✓You can guarantee a healthy pregnancy and a safe birth by paying attention to these suggestions and scheduling regular prenatal appointments. Always remember to look after yourself and your developing child, and don't be afraid to contact your healthcare practitioner if you have any worries or inquiries.

CHAPTER TWO

Why Not Start With A Balanced And Nutritious Diet

Eating a balanced and nutritious diet is vital throughout pregnancy since it gives your growing baby the nutrients they need to thrive and flourish. A good diet can also help you maintain a healthy weight, minimize your risk of pregnancy problems, and boost your general well-being.

So, what should you be eating? A healthy pregnancy diet should include a range of foods from all of the major food groups, including:

Fruits and veggies: Aim to consume at least five servings of fruits and vegetables per day, as these are good sources of vitamins, minerals, and fibre.

Whole grains: Choose whole grain pieces of bread, cereals, and pasta, which give more fibre and nutrients than their refined equivalents.

Lean protein: Include lean meats, poultry, fish, eggs, beans, and tofu in your diet to ensure that you're getting enough protein.

Dairy products: Milk, cheese, and yoghurt are all fantastic sources of calcium, which is vital for having strong bones and teeth.

Healthy fats: Choose sources of healthy fats, such as avocados, nuts, seeds, and

olive oil, to give your body needed fatty acids.

It's also vital to avoid some foods and beverages that can be detrimental to your developing baby, such as:

<u>Raw or undercooked meats and eggs:</u> These might be infected with dangerous microorganisms.

<u>Raw or undercooked seafood:</u> Some varieties of fish can have high levels of mercury, which can be hazardous to your baby's development.

<u>Alcohol:</u> Drinking alcohol during pregnancy can increase your baby's

chances of birth abnormalities and developmental delays.

Caffeine: While moderate caffeine intake is typically considered safe during pregnancy, excessive caffeine consumption can raise your chance of miscarriage.

By eating a balanced and healthy diet, you can offer your growing baby the nutrients they need to develop and flourish. In addition to improving your baby's health, a healthy pregnancy diet can also enhance your health and well-being.

If you're unclear about what to eat during pregnancy, or if you have any unique dietary concerns or restrictions, talk to your healthcare provider or a qualified dietitian. They can provide tailored

counseling and assistance to help you make healthy decisions and ensure that

you and your baby are getting the nutrition
you need.

CHAPTER THREE

Always Stay Hydrated

Staying hydrated throughout pregnancy is critical since it aids in the development of your growing baby and keeps your body running smoothly. When you're pregnant, your body requires more water than usual to aid in the formation of new tissue, the production of amniotic fluid, and the transport of nutrients to your baby. Dehydration during pregnancy can cause a variety of issues such as constipation, exhaustion, headaches, and even preterm labour. To avoid these problems, make sure you drink plenty of water throughout the day.

Most doctors advise pregnant women to drink at least 8-10 glasses of water every day, or more if they exercise or live in a hot region. Fluids can also be obtained via foods such as fruits, vegetables, and soups. If you find it difficult to stay hydrated, try bringing a water bottle with you wherever you go and setting reminders to drink water throughout the day. Drinking fluids with meals or snacks may also be beneficial, as may flavour your water with a piece of lemon or cucumber for extra flavour.

Remember that staying hydrated is a vital aspect of having a healthy pregnancy and can help you feel your best throughout your journey. So drink up and reap the benefits of a hydrated body and baby.

CHAPTER FOUR

Try Regular Exercise

Regular exercise is a crucial aspect of a healthy pregnancy, as it can help you maintain a healthy weight, reduce your risk of pregnancy problems, and enhance your general well-being. Exercise throughout pregnancy can also help prepare your body for labour and delivery, and may even help you recover more rapidly following childbirth.

Most healthcare experts recommend that pregnant women aim for at least 30 minutes of moderate-intensity exercise on most days of the week. This can include exercises such as walking, swimming, prenatal yoga, and low-impact aerobics.

If you're new to exercising or unclear about how to get started, talk to your healthcare physician for individualized assistance and recommendations. They can help you choose the forms of activity that are safe and acceptable for you and your baby and can provide recommendations for staying comfortable and preventing damage.

Remember, while exercising during pregnancy can give numerous benefits, it's crucial to listen to your body and prevent overexertion. Stop exercising if you have any pain, discomfort, or bleeding, and talk to your healthcare practitioner if you have any concerns.

By making fitness a regular part of your pregnancy routine, you may help promote a healthy pregnancy and prepare for the difficulties and joys of motherhood.

CHAPTER FIVE

Take Time To Rest And Sleep.

Because your body is working so hard to support the growth and development of your developing baby, getting enough rest and sleep is crucial throughout pregnancy. Fatigue, mood fluctuations, and even an increased risk of pregnancy issues can result from getting too little or poor quality sleep.

Pregnant women should aim for at least 7-9 hours of sleep every night, or more if necessary, according to the majority of healthcare professionals. Try to maintain a regular sleep schedule and create a cosy sleeping environment to ensure a restful night's sleep.

Avoiding electronic gadgets before bed, maintaining a cool, dark bedroom, and utilizing a supportive pregnancy pillow to ease discomfort and encourage sounder sleep are a few examples of how to do this. To help you relax and de-stress before bed, you could also find it useful to practice relaxation techniques like deep breathing or meditation.

Keep in mind that obtaining enough rest and sleep throughout pregnancy is crucial for both your health and well-being as well as the health and development of your unborn child. So, put relaxation first throughout your pregnancy, and get the rewards of a body and mind that are well-rested.

CHAPTER SIX

Avoid Using Drugs, Alcohol, And Tobacco

It's crucial for the health and growth of your developing child to abstain from drugs, alcohol, and tobacco while you're pregnant. These chemicals may impair the growth, development, and general health of your unborn child and raise the chance of pregnancy issues like preterm labour, low birth weight, and miscarriage.

Speak with your healthcare practitioner if you're having trouble quitting these substances for assistance and advice.

They can provide you with guidance and assistance to help you stop using tobacco, alcohol, and drugs throughout your pregnancy.

Keep in mind that every decision you make during your pregnancy could affect the health and welfare of your unborn child. You can guarantee that your kid has the best start in life and create the conditions for a healthy and happy pregnancy by abstaining from alcohol, tobacco, and drugs.

CHAPTER SEVEN

Consider Antenatal Vitamins

Prenatal vitamins are a crucial component of a healthy pregnancy since they can support the development of your developing child and make sure you're getting the nutrients your body requires to sustain a healthy pregnancy. Prenatal vitamins can help fill any gaps in your diet because they are specifically created to satisfy the special nutritional demands of pregnant women.

Prenatal vitamins should be started by expectant women as soon as they start attempting to conceive or as soon as they learn they are pregnant, according to the majority of healthcare professionals. A combination of vital vitamins and minerals, including folic acid, iron, calcium, and vitamin D, are often included in prenatal vitamins.

Because it can lessen the risk of brain and spine birth abnormalities, folic acid is particularly crucial during the first trimester of pregnancy. Iron is crucial throughout pregnancy as it supports the formation of your unborn child's blood cells.

While prenatal vitamins are crucial, a healthy, balanced diet should still come first. Ensure that you consume a variety of nutrient-dense foods, including fruits, vegetables, whole grains, lean proteins, and dairy products.

Ask your doctor for advice if you're having trouble tolerating prenatal vitamins or aren't sure which brand to pick. They can advise you on how to make prenatal vitamins easier to take and assist you in locating one that suits your needs.

To ensure that your baby receives the nutrients he or she needs to grow and develop, keep in mind that taking prenatal vitamins is an essential component of a successful pregnancy. For a safe and happy pregnancy, prioritize your prenatal vitamins in addition to a nutritious diet and other suggested lifestyle adjustments.

CHAPTER EIGHT

Get Parenting And Childbirth Education.

You can feel more prepared and confident as you handle the trials and rewards of pregnancy and motherhood by educating yourself on birthing and parenting. You can learn about subjects including prenatal care, delivery alternatives, breastfeeding, newborn care, and more with the help of a variety of websites.

Your healthcare practitioner can be a great source of knowledge and direction, and he or she might be able to suggest courses or other resources in your area further your education. A lot of information is also available in books and online, including authoritative websites, blogs, pregnancy and parenting books, and more.

It can also be a terrific chance to interact with other pregnant parents and learn from professionals by enrolling in childbirth and parenting classes. The subjects covered in these sessions might range from prenatal care and pain management methods to newborn care and breastfeeding assistance.

Always keep in mind that every pregnancy and parenting experience is different and that what works for one family may not work for another. As you navigate the thrilling and occasionally daunting world of pregnancy and motherhood, knowing your options and keeping informed may help you feel more confident and in control and assist you in making the right choices for your family and yourself.

CHAPTER NINE

Prepare For The Arrival Of Your Child

Finally! Prepare for the arrival of your child.

Preparing for your baby's arrival may be both thrilling and stressful. There are several things you can do as your due date approaches to help ensure a smooth transition into parenthood.

Make sure you have all of the necessary baby equipment, such as a car seat, cot or bassinet, stroller, and diapering supplies. Make a list of the items you'll need and begin purchasing as soon as possible to guarantee you have everything in time for your baby's arrival.

You should also prepare your home for your new arrival. Creating a secure and comfortable nursery area, baby-proofing your home, and storing up supplies such as diapers, wipes, and baby clothes are all examples of this.

Another critical step is to make arrangements for your baby's care following birth. Choosing a doctor, discussing your birth plan with your healthcare practitioner, and making plans for any necessary support, such as a postpartum doula or lactation consultant, are all examples of things to consider. Finally, remember to take care of yourself during this period. Self-care is essential during pregnancy and after the birth of your child, and it can help you feel your best while you navigate the joys and challenges of motherhood. Getting enough rest, eating a nutritious and balanced diet, and seeking help from loved ones and healthcare providers as needed are all examples of this.

Remember that preparing for your baby's arrival is an ongoing process, and it's perfectly fine to seek assistance and support along the way. You may help ensure a smooth and joyous transition into parenthood with a little forethought and preparation.

CHAPTER TEN

Contact Your Network Of Supporters

When dealing with postpartum mood disorders like depression or anxiety, reaching out to your support network can be extremely important.

They can provide you with a sympathetic ear, offer helpful assistance, and, if necessary, assist in making connections to resources and expert assistance.

It's critical to keep in mind that asking for assistance and support when you require it is acceptable. You don't need to experience pregnancy and parenthood alone. If you're having trouble or need assistance, don't be afraid to seek out your loved ones or your healthcare professionals.

There are various tools available to assist you to connect with other mothers and support services if you don't already have a solid support system. You can get in touch with neighbourhood organizations like parenting clubs or community centres, or you could think about joining online forums or support groups.

Remember that a crucial aspect of becoming a mother is taking care of yourself and getting help when you need it. No matter how big or little your network of supporters may be, don't be afraid to reach out to them. They can give you the love and support you need to survive while assisting you in navigating the ups and downs of pregnancy and parenting.

CONCLUSION

The health of the expectant mother and the developing child should come first. You now have the knowledge and advice you need to confidently navigate pregnancy and parenting as a result of this handbook. These ten suggestions can help you prepare for childbirth and parenthood, manage the physical and emotional changes of pregnancy, and make decisions that are best for you and your baby.

Keep in mind that every pregnancy is different from the next, so what works for one woman might not work for another. It's crucial to pay attention to your body's signals and speak with your doctor if you have any worries or inquiries. They can provide you with individualized guidance and assistance to ensure that your pregnancy is healthy and pleasant.

Don't forget to have fun when travelling in addition to following these 10 guidelines! A period of exciting change and transformation in your life, pregnancy can bring you new joys, difficulties, and experiences. Spend time bonding with your developing child, acknowledging milestones, and appreciating the love and support of your loved ones.

We hope that this guide has given you useful information and resources to support a healthy pregnancy and happy motherhood. Take care of yourself and your kid, get help when you need it, and take pleasure in this unique period of your life. Best wishes for a joyful and healthy pregnancy and the rest of your life!